NURSING
FROM
WITHIN

NURSING *from* WITHIN

A Fresh Alternative to Putting Out Fires and Self-Care Workarounds

ELIZABETH SCALA

PRAISE FOR NURSING FROM WITHIN

"Elizabeth Scala's message is compelling for nurses who are seeking ways to become happier, healthier, and more inspired about their work. In addition to her enthusiastic vision of the "Art of Nursing" she shares her heartfelt personal story, many familiar experiences that colleagues can relate to and offers several activities that are easy to incorporate in the day to day stressful realities of professional practice". -Beth Boynton, Author of "Confident Voices"

"A smart, concise, fun and above all informational book on being smarter about how to work as a nurse. This book is a must-have for anyone who is a nurse, wants to become a nurse and/or who supports nurses". -Nicole M. Brown, Author of "N is for Nurse"

"Nursing from Within" is an inspiring read that offers a diagnosis of today's care giving challenges and a prescription for liberating the most powerful healing medicine known: Love.

Elizabeth artfully shares her personal journey of spiritual awakening. Along the way, you'll learn how to apply methods and insights that can re-fire professional and personal passion for living. Even more important, you'll learn the secret to discovering ever deeper feelings of happiness and wellbeing.

As a stress mastery practitioner, I will be recommending Elizabeth's book to medical professional and other clients. You'll find a wealth of wisdom offered in this delightful book. I highly recommend it". -Stephen W. Carter, MA, CHt

"Drawing from her own life experiences, Elizabeth Scala compassionately demonstrates how her fellow nurses can experience inner peace and joy in a profession known for uncertainty and heightened stress levels". -Nat Couropmitree, Author of "The Giving Person's Self-Care Guide"

"A brave and visionary book. Elizabeth Scala presents the problems in Nursing but focuses on the transformation in thought that has to be accomplished before we can heal ourselves, our patients and our system. I loved it". -Carol Gino RN, MA, Author of several best-selling books including "The Nurse's Story"

"This innovative and fresh approach is a brilliant plan to shift the nursing profession towards real health and healing. Elizabeth's passion and vulnerability as she shares her story and teachings are beyond inspiring". - Betty Louise, CPCC, and Author of "Healing with Pleasure Medicine: Unearthing the Beautiful, Sensual, and Sexual You"

"New, seasoned or disabled nurse.....this book is a gift for you! Learn to "show up" joyful.... heart open... have fun... and "choose" to walk unique, new paths in life and nursing". - Donna Carol Maheady, EdD, ARNP, and Author of "Leave No Nurse Behind: Nurses working with disAbilities"

"Nursing is never easy. We leave our shift physically exhausted and emotionally spent. We get up the next day and do it all over again. Why?! Because we make a difference. Elizabeth Scala explores the adventures we have all had and shows us ways to renew our love for nursing and care for our own body and soul. This is a MUST read for every nurse". -Kathy Quan RN, BSN, PHN, Author of several books including "The Everything New Nurse Book"

"In clinical practice, scientific knowledge, expert skills, and sound judgment are essential, but they're not a complete picture of the consummate nurse. The missing puzzle piece is described in this profound book. Scala elucidates a path to practicing as your authentic self and offers sophisticated ways to cope with stress and burnout. This book is exciting and necessary". -Tilda Shalof RN, BScN, Author of "A Nurse's Story."

"At a time in the health care industry where change is rapid and daunting, Elizabeth Scala offers keen insights and inspiration to those who follow in her footsteps as a nursing professional. This book is worth the read for nurses of all disciplines". -Brian Luke Seaward, Ph.D. Author of "Stand Like Mountain, Flow Like Water"

"Personable, accessible, and very refreshing; not to mention helpful. Elizabeth's written to her audience in a way that brings them directly in and creates trust, obviously writing from experience and a deep desire to bring change. I've worked with nurses over the past 15 years providing Reiki Training and Stress Management techniques and I think this book is a very valuable resource". -Stephanie Shelburne, NhD, PhDc, CMT

"A candid problem - solution model, offering proven holistic strategies to enrich and uplift nurses and nursing". -Annette Tersigni RN, Founder of YogaNursing®, Author of "The Richest Woman In Babylon And Manhattan"

"Consider taking a chance with this book. You might learn something new or reaffirm what's already been working for you. The last two chapters were a homerun for me". -Kimberly Raquel Ward BSN RN, Author of "What They Didn't Teach You Or I In Nursing School: Lessons Learned Outside The Classroom."

"An insightful, life-changing book for any nurse who neglects their own self-care i.e. most of us. It offers thoughtful, practical advice you can start using right now. All nurses should read it!" - Allie Wilson RN, Editor of 'Wellbeing for Nurses Magazine'

Alicia Forest, more than my coach: my guide, my teacher and my inspiration. Thank you for your continued support, the endless resources and your authentic intuition. Through our work together, I have become unstuck, finally moving myself forward out of the limiting patterns that held me back. Your caring, yet forward nudge to either go for it or throw it all in, moved me out of fear into confidence. Your belief in me has gifted me with the most important lesson of all: I now believe in and value myself. I am grateful you choose to show up as your true self each day, as you instill that same courage in all of us that you coach to do the same.

TABLE OF CONTENTS

FOREWORD

Nurses are often so busy caring for other people; they neglect to care for themselves. Many are exhausted, discouraged, and burning out.

Nearly twenty years ago I quit my "day job" as a practicing nurse and studied to become a professional speaker and author, in order to inspire my beleaguered colleagues and teach them tools to care for themselves while they care for everybody else. When I wrote both editions of *Chicken Soup for the Nurse's Soul*, I offered them the healing power of stories from their fellow nurses. In my presentations and seminars, I gave nurses strategies to care for their minds, bodies, and spirits *every day.* Even though I teased them that I hadn't taught them anything they didn't already know, they reported being transformed by my messages of self-care. (That's how desperate they were for the information!)

They said they wanted more...that they wished the entire hospital and all of their coworkers could practice the tools of self-care. At their urging, I developed the 12 month initiative *Self Care for HealthCare™, Your Guide to Physical, Mental and Spiritual Health* , where everyone on the healthcare team engages in the same self-care strategies every month. With videos, workbooks and weekly motivations, I teach them simple ways to eat, exercise and sleep in healthy amounts to care for themselves physically. I share the science and techniques to care for themselves mentally every day with deep breathing, relaxation, positive thinking, laugher and forgiveness. And I coach them on how and why to connect with their Higher Power daily.

Elizabeth Scala's *Nursing from Within* offers similar approaches and application of these universal truths. Elizabeth also noted that her fellow nurses were giving so much love and compassion to their patients, that their minds were taxed, bodies drained, and spirits tired. I knew her work was brilliant when it so closely paralleled mine.

Nursing from Within not only gives strategies and practices to care for ourselves physically, mentally and spiritually, but adjusts our mindsets to approach self-care from a new and healthy perspective. Elizabeth guides readers to a change their viewpoints and perceptions and she helps nurses make the inner shift needed to better maneuver the challenges of practicing nursing today.

Both Elizabeth and I have seen the age-old issues and problems continue to resurface throughout our careers. Healthcare givers often try to fix these challenges with the same mindsets that created them. In this book, she offers a fresh perspective of solutions that work; she empowers nurses to create health and happiness in their own lives. Elizabeth shows readers how to shift their inner perspective so they can enjoy their outer environments, no matter how stressful they may be, by using the power of their minds to make a conscious choice to improve their health, career and lives.

I respect Elizabeth's courage to be vulnerable. By allowing her authentic self to shine throughout Nursing from Within, her work inspires nurses to enjoy their careers on a daily basis. Elizabeth's energy and enthusiasm for the nursing profession is truly contagious.

Every person, hospital and organization I speak to agrees that nurses of strong mind, body and spirit deliver better patient care, which results in better outcomes, satisfactions scores, and ultimately reimbursements.

The answer to our healthcare challenges today lies in caring for the nurse.

Nursing from Within confirms that belief...that fact. This book will transform caregivers from the inside out as it is driven by principles, grounded in scientific theory, and backed by quantum physics and the laws of energy. Elizabeth's specific daily practices will help nurses enjoy clarity, confidence, vision, and empowerment so that they can perform their best in the healing art of nursing in healthy, happy, and holistic environments.

LeAnn Thieman, Nurse, Author, Hall of fame Speaker

Author *Chicken Soup for the Nurse's Soul, Chicken Soup for a the Nurse's Soul, Second Dose, Chicken Soup for the Caregiver's Soul,* and *Self Care for HealthCare™, Your Guide to Physical, Mental and Spiritual Health.* www.LeAnnThieman.com

PREFACE

I wrote this book for the nursing profession, one that I have become more fond of than I could have ever imagined. This book is for the individual nurse reader, for through our own authentic empowerment we are able to make epic shifts.

Healthcare is experiencing major change, some of it exceptionally healthy, while other aspects could be perceived as tumultuous. I believe that nursing is the profession which makes up the healthcare system. As the eyes and ears of around the clock care, we embody the professional backbone of our cultural well-being.

It is my intention that you read this book with an open heart and a beginner's mind. Some of the concepts may be familiar and instead of nodding them off as "I already know", ask yourself this question:

Am I a living role model of what I know?

Other aspects of this book may be foreign, new and exciting to you, or unknown and thus, a bit scary. Reading gently with a sense of unconditional love can open many doors for you. The book can be read once through and then pieces that call to your spirit can be visited again for even greater digestion and detail.

So that you are further supported, I have also taken the time to create a complementary workbook that is meant to accompany this book. If you enjoy the reading and want to take things a step further, I encourage you to proactively engage in the workbook exercises.

Finally, I thank you for being a nurse. The profession of nursing has made me feel so humbled, honored and full of dedicated joy. It is wonderful to share this beautiful role of service with you.

Happy reading!

INTRODUCTION

I didn't really want to be a nurse. In fact, I used to curse my mother for pushing me into the accelerated nursing program. I hated the courses and struggled through Chemistry, Pathophysiology and Pharmacology.

While I didn't exactly know '*what I wanted to be when I grew up*', the four women who stood in the living room of my senior year college apartment sure filled in the blanks for me. Even though I despised hospitals and felt totally uncomfortable around sick people, my mother, two new roommates and one of their moms (a nursing instructor at my university) planned my entire life for me that hot and humid move-in day.

"*Well, what does Elizabeth want to* do *when she finishes college*?" Celeste's mom asked me (or was it that she asked my mom?).

"*She doesn't know yet,*" my mother answered in quick exasperation before I could even offer my ideas of graduate school for a master's degree in psychology.

"*I've got an idea! She could do the accelerated nursing program. She already has most of her credits and there are just a few requirements she'd have to catch up on. If she is so far ahead right now* (which I was since I had taken so many advanced courses in high school and summer classes at college every year) *she could just jump right in and be done in no time.*"

"*And she could be a psychiatric nurse. Since she's going to have a psych degree, then that's the type of nurse she will be,*" my other roommate chimed in.

For the next 15 minutes or so (what felt like a painful eternity to me), the four of them discussed exactly how I would get it done. My roommates, both of whom were on target to graduate that May from the traditional nursing program, were extremely helpful in designing the rest of my life for me.

Well there you have it- how I became a nurse.

My story might be viewed as the exception to the rule since I've heard that so many nurses have felt 'called' into our profession. My recent work has led me to survey hundreds of nurses over the course of several entrepreneurial activities. As recently as last summer I asked dozens of nurses the question: "*Why is it that you became a nurse?*"

"*I got really sick when I was in grammar school and I'll never forget the nurse who took care of me. I knew from that day on I wanted to be just like her.*"

"*I hurt myself at summer camp and this beautiful angel came to my rescue. I now realize she was a nurse and I knew I wanted to help other people, just as she helped me.*"

There were so many other responses, similar to those above. From having a sick family member and watching the compassionate nurse ease their pain, to the honor that comes with having nearly every relative they can remember work as a nurse and just knowing that nursing was the professional course they too, would take. Nurses often answer a 'calling'; knowing from a very early age that this is what they're meant to do.

So then why is nursing in such turmoil? How come we have an army of caregivers who struggle to care for themselves? Why do so many nurses, good nurses- no, *great* nurses- want to leave the bedside? What is it about nursing that makes it so challenging?

This book is very simple; some may find it so simple that in fact, it becomes a challenge. Over the course of the pages that follow, I plan to outline for you the problems faced by today's nurse, offer a straightforward solution to our challenges and share with you proven and effective strategies for creating epic shifts.

I am really excited to help you, your colleagues and our profession as a whole. I believe in nursing and what we do. While I may not have gone into nursing knowing I wanted to be a nurse, the nurse inside of me has come out in a really big way.

1

Nursing is Hard Work

"Medicine sometimes snatches away health,
sometimes gives it." –Ovid

It's New Year's Day. I'm kind of tired because well, let's just be honest, I'm still a party girl and I was out late last night. We're standing in the day room, the four of us, doing mid-day report. "Why the day room?" you might ask. "Why not sit down, grab a snack and share report in the break room?"

Great question, but since many of you reading this book are probably nurses, I'm certain you know the answer. We're short-staffed and don't even have enough coverage to watch the seven patients who are on constant observation (I'm a psych nurse, remember).

At least we have a great team today. I'm in charge, Eddie did rounds with the physicians and Emma and Julie are two of our best new nurses to the unit. Yes, we've got two new graduate nurses on with me and one other nurse. We're at full capacity and the ED keeps calling, asking when they can send the new admission up.

The four of us huddle, regrouping and trying to figure out how we might make it through the next eight hours, if any of us will get to eat and which one of us may have to stay late because- oh yes, that's right- the evening shift is short too.

After the team breaks from the mid-shift updates, I head to the supply room. I've got to change the bag of Normal Saline in room 402 and Ms. Jones asked for some new footie's. Well, wouldn't you know? We're out of Normal Saline and the only pair of footie's left will fit a much larger sized male patient.

To top it all off, as I'm in the supply room cursing at the Central Store's Department I hear yelling in the hallway. "Great," I think to myself. "A patient's going off... let's see who it is this time."

When I exit the closet I am in total shock. No, it's not a manic patient screaming about their medication. It isn't even our dementia patient in 419. It's one of the ladies on our support staff and she is yelling at the security guard who watches over our unit. "Wonderful," I mutter. As charge nurse, guess who gets to figure this mess out?

I could go on- and on- and even on again. But, you get my drift. You've been there. You know how it ends. Driving home close to tears; exhausted and drained, you can't even see the road. Then flopping onto the couch, shuttering at the fact you have to get up in five hours and do it all over again (yes, I was the lucky one who got to stay late).

Nursing is hard work. It's physically demanding, emotionally draining and doesn't get easier with time or age. In the next three chapters I'll share with you some of the struggles we face, both inside and outside of our control. Now you might be thinking, "Heck, I could write those chapters myself." And yes, while I do agree, I'm going to describe them here in more global detail than just the issues presented to you and me.

Ready? Let's get to work.

First, I'd like to break down the challenges a single nurse can face on any given day into three categories. (Now I know there are probably many more difficulties a nurse may face than I have time to share here in this book, -in fact one could probably write an entire Encyclopedia and call it 'Nurse Problems'- but I'll do my best to provide an over-arching picture and, using your life experience, you can fill in the rest).

The three major groupings that nurse struggles fit into are the following:

- Self (you know, those types of challenges that one person can experience)
- Others (those socially oriented issues that have to do with people around you)
- And global/environmental (some of those bigger picture or demographic themes of our times)

Now that being said, let's go through each of them in a bit more detail.

Self

As I said above, nursing is hard work. It's physically demanding. It's exhausting. You know as well as I do that sometimes when you leave that job you feel like you were run over by a tractor trailer.

You might be scheduled to work 4 twelve hour shifts in a row, night ones too (when you're a day person). You work weekends, holidays, on calls and over time. The end is never in sight.

Even when you're off, and I know you know what I'm talking about (I can feel it as I type this sentence), you're thinking about work, bringing work home with you, dreading going back to work and wondering if work will call. Have you ever gotten to the place where every time the phone rings you cringe; thinking it might be work calling and asking you for help?

Nursing is a labor-intensive job. You're lifting patients, on your feet all day, and running around the hospital. Maybe your back aches or your feet hurt, but after long years of experience, the job has taken its toll on your body.

Just the very nature of our job, its go-go-go all of the time. There is no 'sitting down'. We eat standing up, if at all. You can't seem to catch a break. I know I've said it a few times now, but I'll say it once more: nursing is hard work.

Being a nurse can have you feeling like your emotions are on a roller coaster ride. One day you're angry with the job; the next your elated at how rewarding it can be. At home you don't know whether to laugh or cry. You're giving so much love and compassion of yourself to your patients that at times you feel totally numb.

The mind is taxed. The body is drained. The spirit is tired.

Others

While nursing is hard, you know how challenging it can be to work as a team. Even with our best intentions at raising morale, leveling the playing field and treating colleagues with respect, sometimes the 'other people' in our professional lives can get in our way.

Not just the coworkers- but the patients. Think about it. How often is your unit running at or above full capacity? Isn't it all too common these days that you're functioning over-census? And don't get me started on how we calculate patient hours per day and the fact that these measurements have gone out of style, let's stick to the topic.

Patients are also getting older, sicker and much more acute. With the wonderful advancements in medicine we're no longer seeing as many people pass away from chronic conditions. Don't get me wrong, it's fabulous that our loved ones and family members get to stick around longer than they used to, but what does this do to the nurse? The ones taking care of these patients are now seeing patients living with lengthier disease processes and there are lots of new struggles that arise with that.

Besides the patients, you've got your team. And OY! Just writing the word team I am feeling some of you shudder.

We all know the slogans and catch-phrases that are used with how we relate to each other in the nursing world, so I won't even bring those up here, but working with a team full of unique and varying personalities is hard work. And it's not just the nursing staff.

Oh- I opened a can of worms on that one didn't I? Interactions with ancillary departments, support staff and even the providers can leave us feeling exasperated and demoralized. Going to our supervisor, peer support team or manager can help- or not?

Managers mean well, but they have their own set of challenges. You want a manager who is visible, approachable and willing to help out, but they've got people breathing down their necks too. Between emails, meetings and the reports they have to review, submit and beautify, they're also short on time!

Leadership does not seem to know what managers know; managers think they know what nurses know; no one seems to be happy with anyone. The 'team' feel that we all hope and dream for sometimes gets lost in the shuffle.

It is no one's fault at all. It is the nature of the beast. The very beast that we call nursing. Taking care of patients, taking care of our staff and taking care of each other can just be plain difficult.

Global

We've covered our own personal hardships; we've tackled the teammate strife; now, onto the bigger picture. Remember, as I shared above, this list is not all inclusive. One could spend an entire book on all of the adversity nurses face, but let's be honest, that's no fun. I want to get to the solution and strategies, remember? So without further ado, I present to you the things outside of our control.

It's a moot point, since we've been living this reality for some time now, but the economic situation doesn't help the pressures placed upon nursing. We're forced to cut our staffing, eliminate perks such as education and indirect time and work on shoelace string budgets. Nursing is the biggest group that makes up healthcare systems numbers so when they need to cut down on costs, guess where they turn?

I discussed the advances of medicine when I was speaking about our aging patient population, yet in addition to these wonderful new treatments and therapies comes the age of technology. Documentation goes electronic and charting becomes time-consuming and obsessive. There's no time with the patient as every nurse has his or her face glued to a computer screen. That healing touch of patient care is gone and, no matter where you work or who you work for, as a nurse, you feel it.

As technology takes over, things become faster and response times shorter. People expect you to do more with less. Forget about critical thinking and developing skills, who has time to ponder these days? Information is overloaded and we just can't handle being 'on' all of the time, but we are.

The economic climate, technological advancements and constant connectivity via computers and mobile devices creates so many interlocked network webs it's no wonder our patients (and ourselves?) can't navigate the healthcare system. Patient care falls through the cracks. Family members get confused on what to do next. Caregivers (that's us) get exhausted from this ever changing labyrinth of ideas, people and information.

Yikes, I'm getting tired just visualizing it all. OK, I think that's enough. Sure, we can continue to delve deeper into these personal and professional issues, but really, who wants to? And further, you know it already! You work and live it every day.

So, let's move on to the next phase of the issue: the way things have always been done.

2

Time for a Paradigm Shift

"If your actions inspire others to dream more,
learn more, do more and become more,
you are a leader." -John Quincy Adams

Night shift on a psychiatric unit can be an interesting one. Sometimes we joke that everything depends on the moon or the time of the month. Would the patients sleep tonight? Will we get an admission that needs locked door seclusion? It was like walking around on eggshells, not wanting to wake any of the manic patients that finally fell asleep up.

"Don't wake them up" the lead tech tells me.

"Why? He's ordered for vital signs every four hours. He's here to detox off of alcohol and pills. We've got to wake him up."

"Don't wake him up. We don't do four-hour vital signs at night. We can wait an hour or two and do it close to the start of day shift. That's just how we do it at night here."

I'm still new to the unit, heck I'm new to charge. I've only been off of orientation two months and tonight when I came in there was no one else to run charge. The nurse I'm working with is newer than me! You can imagine my dilemma as I stand there, staring dumb-founded and unsettled.

'That's the way it's done around here' is a term I hear a lot in my unit, a term I hear a lot in nursing. In fact, it's a term I hear a lot in this hospital.

If I listen to 'how it's always been done' I go along with a staff member with greater longevity on this unit than I have. I make an ally and therefore have a work environment that's easier for me to handle. But if I go along with her, the patient care is compromised. This patient is here in alcohol withdrawal for goodness sake. Not only have I studied the books and passed my medication exam, I have a family member I've seen in real life have alcohol withdrawal. I know what it can do to the body.

If I don't listen to her, I potentially make an enemy on this floor and this particular tech; well she seems to run this unit. Do I dare piss her off?

I make the nursing decision, go with my gut on this one and deal with the consequences later.

"That may be how it's always done at night, but that's not how I do it. I'm going in to get his vital signs and you can go down and do Mr. Jones' vitals in 313. Thank you."

Yes, it may have been hard for me to fit in to my unit initially, but I chose to do what was right by the patient and over time, this tech, and all of the other staff on my unit, came to respect me.

It's hard when you're new. There's a way things have always been done and then there's the way you choose to provide nursing care. It's up to you, but I'm sure you've experienced it too.

I've actually never been one to do it 'how it's always been done'. I challenge the status quo, do what's best for myself and those involved and often make choices that go against the grain. Maybe that's why I couldn't stay on my unit, haven't been able to stay at one particular job for longer than 4 years or the reason I never ran with any one particular crowd. Doing things 'the way they've always been done' doesn't spark my interest.

Yet if you're a nurse like me, I bet you've heard one of the following phrases:

"That's how it's always been done."

"That's the way we do it here."

These are the very phrases that have gotten us into so much trouble, those which keep our profession down and make it hard for us to rise to the top of healthcare. These types of phrases create limited thinking and lessen our chances for successful, creative solutions.

There are several pieces to this concept and I'd like to go through them one-by-one in this chapter. In the pages that follow we're going to cover: *the problem-solving approach; Band-Aids that don't fix things; root cause thinking and using the same mindset for both problem and solution.*

It sounds like a lot but it's fairly straight-forward and going through each piece-by-piece will allow it to all make sense in the end. So let's go.

Problem-Solving Approach

Let's look at the medical model for a moment, the model that our healthcare system is based around here in the West. A patient comes to us with a concern, a discomfort. Something is wrong. What usually follows? We ask a bunch of questions, gathering background data, and then we look for a solution to fix the problem. Our goal is to treat and cure, making things all better so that we can send the patient on their merry way.

The same can hold true for our nursing projects, workgroups, meetings and academia. There's something wrong so as nurses we get together, have a meeting and talk about how we are going to fix it.

Maybe the budget needs to be cut or our communication with the dietary department has to improve, whatever the case may be, we sit around in our meeting rooms and talk about the problem. I know you've experienced this before. I'm hearing all of the time about how nurses are involved in one too many meetings per day.

So after we discuss the problem ad nauseam, we look back on how we've fixed things before, either in the same case or in similar situations, and we start to offer possible solutions. We talk and talk, and talk some more, until we come up with an agreed upon answer.

Problem equals solution. Solution will fix what is wrong. Right? Not so much.

Band-Aids Don't Fix Things

What happens when you get a cut? If it's bad enough, you usually cover it up with a band-aid, right? Now does the band-aid heal the cut? No. As a nurse, I'm sure you can agree that the band-aid itself only covers up the cut skin so that beneath the band-aid healing can happen.

I've seen this in healthcare as well.

If someone isn't performing up to par at their job, instead of doing something about the underlying cause, we talk around the problem. We cover it up.

14

Maybe we give them other duties to perform. The tasks that they were not getting to are farmed out and given to someone else. Maybe they get moved into another role, but do they receive what they really need which could mean more education, a good hard look at if they are a fit for the company or a deeper delve into what's really going on? Not necessarily.

Putting a band-aid over an issue without really getting to the underlying cause of things does more harm than good.

Nurses are great at this. In fact, I believe the technical term is called a 'nursing workaround'. You know the drill. We find something wrong and instead of getting at the underlying cause, we work around it.

I think, and I'm sure you would agree, that the number one thing they didn't teach you in nursing school that comes in handy the *most* is our ability to work around a problem, finding a solution so that we can continue on with our jobs.

This can get us into trouble. In fact it has. Nurses are often faced with something that sounds like this: 'Oh you nurses, you're so good at fixing things. We're sure you can handle it.' People start to perceive that we can handle anything and then expect us to do less with more. In fact, I believe that we've created some of our patient-nurse staffing ratio issues ourselves. Organizational leadership has figured out that nurses are MacGyver's in scrubs. We can, do and will fix anything.

One last problem with us fixing things at face value and not really solving underlying issues: we find ourselves working to less than our degrees. Central stores can't get us a supply; we walk down and get it. Intradepartmental mail doesn't have the staff to sort letters; nurses find themselves stuffing mailboxes. Supportive administrative staff calls out; guess who's answering the unit telephones? We continue to work around, helping everyone out but ourselves, and we wonder why nursing is doing everyone else's job?

Root Cause Thinking

As I've alluded to above, what's really needed to improve and heal a situation is getting at the underlying cause of it. What's really going on here?

Medicine has become so specialized these days. We have providers specializing in every single ailment, body part and unique situation out there. When a patient has a problem they are often seen by a whole host of specialists and each person's assessment, plan and treatment could be different.

What happened to whole person healing?

In a more holistic model we know that everything is interrelated. A troubling situation or stressful experience could have occurred, and because of the way you perceive it, a stressor may crop up in the body-mind-spirit system. Then your holding onto that stressor creates tension and blockage in certain areas of the body. The symptoms that present themselves are not just a depiction of the physical illness. They are so much more!

In fact, physical symptoms are actually the end processes of what's really going on with the patient. When an issue gets as far as manifesting itself in the form of physical disease symptoms, the person has actually been struggling with the concern much longer than anyone realizes. Instead of treating symptoms, we should be tracing them back to the root cause of the experience.

Linking this back to nursing, again we cannot just look at the surfaced 'problem' and fix it at that level. We've got to go deeper and deeper, and probably even deeper, if we want to get to the root cause of things. If we want to make any kind of significant and sustainable change, we've got to get to the underlying circumstances.

Sitting in a meeting and discussing an issue that your workgroup is having with another ancillary department won't create lasting change. In fact, coming up with an answer to a communication issue with another policy or protocol won't do a thing at all. We've got to get at the root cause of the situation and find a way to heal the entire process, from beginning to end.

The Same Mindset for Both Problem and Solution

"We can't solve problems by using the same kind of thinking we used when we created them." - Albert Einstein

All of what I've shared above speaks to Einstein's ingenious words.

To use the problem-solving, band-aid approach in nursing is taking our very minds that have created our issues and challenging circumstances and using those same tools to try to fix things. We won't get anywhere. We just won't.

I have watched this in action.

I have seen, observed and been involved with meetings at the various jobs I've held in my life. I am a member of a nursing association. I have colleagues who work in both the clinical and academic setting. I am all over the internet reading articles, involved in forums and take part in nursing-based discussion groups.

We are running in circles, people. It's no wonder we're feeling as though we're on a hamster wheel, too tired to get off of it. If we keep this up we're going to be no farther along than we were 20,

30, even 50 years ago. In fact we may move backwards before we leap forwards.

And that is just what it may take, a leap. A leap of faith. A leap of something new and different. A leap of fresh perspective. A leap of something innovative, creative and fresh that will help our profession survive, thrive and grow.

Let's talk a bit more about this leap in the next chapter, as this image of leaping may not be so far-fetched after we discuss something I've learned about called the Funnel of Limitation.

3

Break Free from Limitation

*"I'm not telling you it's going to be easy,
I'm telling you it's going to be worth it."* -Art Williams

I used to be the one in our unit to arrange our monthly happy hours. I'd pick a new place, which usually had good food and drink specials, and was always in another part of town. We'd all save the date and head out after work, one weekday a month, to get together, have some fun and let loose.

Well, was it fun that we actually had?

The happy hour would start off nice. Simple, casual, lots of laughter and not so much discussion about work. As the happy 'hour' dragged on and one-by-one the leadership members would leave to go home, our happiness of happy hour would dwindle down.

We'd start in on work.

We'd talk about all of the things wrong with our unit, complain and vent non-stop about our colleagues and just get plain nasty with gossip and negativity. To those of you who worked with me, I'm sorry if you didn't feel or see it this way. This is how the monthly happy hours went for me.

I was the one being negative. I was the one gossiping. I was the one bringing up each and every single thing wrong with the workplace.

Even when we tried to change the subject and shift to something more positive and light, I found myself circling back to the problems with work.

Yes, I was a leader on my unit, but as I reflect back on it, what was I leading my unit and colleagues to?

This story is a perfect example of what I've learned about from Dr. Robert Anthony and his teachings on the Funnel of Limitation.

Dr. Robert Anthony has worked as a psychotherapist trained in all forms of Energy Therapy including Neuro-linguistic programming (NLP), Thought Field Therapy (TFT), Tapas Acupressure Technique (TAT), and Emotional Freedom Technique (EFT). Dr. Anthony's work has focused on identifying, describing and then teaching us how the mind holds the ultimate key to peak personal performance in all areas. (I personally have benefited from multiple audio and print programs that Dr.

Anthony has created and you can find these in the appendix of this book).

In one particular program that I took with Dr. Anthony, he described something that he, which is called the Funnel of Limitation. Let's talk about this a bit here as it relates to our nursing practice and profession.

Picture the shape of a funnel. It's cone-like with the narrowest part being at the bottom and the top opening up in a circular fashion.

Now what Dr. Anthony suggests is that we can imagine we are all placed inside of this funnel shape. There are people packed into the funnel, both at the bottom and near the top. Where you are and those people surrounding you in the funnel, both shape and impact your experiences.

What you want to do is reach your personal peak potential and eventually get yourself out of the Funnel of Limitation. If you find yourself near the bottom of the funnel, what's happening is you are being held down by the limitations of both yourself and those who are near the bottom with you.

You look around, left to right or in front of and behind you, and you are surrounded by others who are similar to you. The people near you, at the bottom of the funnel, share your same challenges and afflictions. They go through the same struggles and experience similar dramas and traumas.

Even if you wanted to get out you may find you have an extremely difficult time because as you look around, at those people around you, you find an overwhelming sense of impossibility. You are literally drowning in the funnel of limitations. Even if you try to make a simple change in your life that will help you move towards the top of the funnel, the beliefs, perceptions and attitudes of those around you will severely impact and limit your chances of success.

Now let's take this analogy and apply it to nursing.

What is nursing? It is a large group of people, at this time predominately still female-dominated, who are in close proximity to each other.

We have gone through similar training; we hold similar values; we work for a common cause. We work in close proximity, often in groups and are often surrounded by colleagues and co-workers. We're placed on teams and rely heavily on each other to get the job done.

We also typically travel in packs. We join nurse's associations. We go to nursing conferences. We attend meetings within the nursing profession that solve nursing problems.

What if all of this nursing 'togetherness' has created a tribal think?

Do we not suffer from similar challenges? Couldn't you call up any nurse that you know right now and vent something awful to them and what would happen? Most likely they would completely understand, maybe even have gone through it themselves.

Aren't nursing terms, phrases and language so universal that we've created some form of group think?

It is possible that nursing, the entire profession as we know it today, is stuck. Bogged down from the energy that is created within the funnel. Looking left and right, turning around or glancing above us- who do we see? What do we hear? Where do we go for answers?

We hear the same things, talk about the same things and live the same things.

While nursing has come a very long way in terms of scientific skills and critical thinking, can we say the same thing for our own personal and professional evolvement as a whole? Are we developing in a way that will help us to thrive and move forward as a group? Or is the mindset of 'this is how it's always been done' keeping us stuck in the funnel of nursing limitation?

In the following chapters of this book I will encourage you to do something totally radical.

Be you.

There is no way we will change nursing, uplift the profession, empower ourselves by doing the same things we've always done. Keeping with the problem-solving approach and fixing our issues with the same group that got us here just won't work anymore.

Now is a time for change. But change must come from the inside out. To change the group, each individual part has to shift. To be a happy, healthy and holistically satisfied group, we must start one nurse at a time.

No, this won't be simple. It will require a transformation. Change doesn't happen overnight and it's not always easy or comfortable. Change has to come from within. You have to want it more than you feel safe and cozy with staying the same. In the words of my coach, Alicia Forest,

"Desire's got to be greater than doubt."

So, if you're ready to leap out of the Funnel of Limitation, letting go of the old way, continue on with me as I'm about to share with you the tools to get you where you want to go.

4

A Blend of Masculine and Feminine Energies

"I am of certain convinced that the greatest heroes are those who do their duty in the daily grind of domestic affairs whilst the world whirls as a maddening dreidel."
— *Florence Nightingale*

There are times in nursing when you act beyond the monitors, lab results and scientific readings. Thankfully, as a brand new nurse I listened to my gut one of these times.

I was working with my preceptor one night shift towards the end of my orientation. We were down in our seven bed detoxification unit. I was on a stretch of nights so we had been there for the past two.

One man, who routinely was an early riser, did not get up out of bed at his usual five thirty in the morning. While we had just done his four am vital signs, I had this strange feeling that something was not right and that we should check on him again.

His blood pressure and heart rate readings weren't due again for another two hours or so, but this man was with us for detoxification from alcohol and I knew how severe that type of withdrawal could be.

So I insisted. I reported to my preceptor that something just did not feel right to me and that even though his four am vital sign check was all within normal limits, I was going in to check on his blood pressure and heart rate again.

Good thing I did! His reading had sky-rocketed. Now this was almost ten years ago as I write this passage so I don't have the exact numbers for you, but they were bad.

I immediately went to my preceptor and we paged the doctor on call. We got this man an additional dose of his medication and avoided a near crisis. I felt so grateful that I had not only my nursing skills that night, but also my gut feeling that something was not right.

Sure, we can use the machines and monitors all day long, but that night shift taught me that in addition to the science of nursing practice I also had to feel into my art of being a nurse.

Nursing has often been referred to as a beautiful blend of art and science. We've got the technical skills, the critical thinking, and the analytical brain. We're logical beings, looking for ways to help, heal and cure. As we've discussed earlier, we're great at assessing the situation, coming up with a solution and evaluating our work.

So what about the 'art'? That human touch and healing connection our nursing pioneers envisioned for us as they set out healing and helping with purposeful, soulful work. What about the presence of simply being a nurse? Has that gotten lost in the shuffle of our day-to-day affairs? Affairs, which, any one of you reading knows, have become busied, buried and overwhelming in nature.

I mentioned my surveying and polling of nurses during the introduction of this book, but let me touch on it in brief again. I've often asked the nurses in my network: what are some of the struggles you face in doing your job, the very career you value above (at times) your own health and well-being?

In unison I hear a resounding theme: the science of nursing.

We've got the computerized charting and electronic medical record. We're expected to get patients in and out in what seems like no time at all. We're accused of having our faces buried in the screen all day, but we've got protocols, policies and procedures to follow. It's task after task after task. We're so rushed that even the critical thinking skills which nursing was founded upon, the very asset we take such pride in as a profession, are being lost on our newer generation of nurses.

How can we focus amidst all of this chaos? How can we find calm (and time) in our busy shift?

Well you may not love what I'm about to share with you, but I want to introduce another aspect of science, a novel approach to nursing science, that can help us reconnect with the art.

Before I do, let's briefly review one of the current models that our healthcare system is working from, as a means to compare it to another model that I'd like to suggest will help us rekindle the art of nursing.

Newtonian Physics

One year I had the privilege to sit on a panel of healthcare providers at a Reiki conference (further information on Reiki to follow in upcoming chapters and more resources in the Appendix of this book). A comment was made by an audience member that will help us get through our journey of scientific thought and theory.

"In healthcare we've got all of the tools. We're educated about the body. We've got the information about illness, disease, and what behaviors can help

prevent it. We 'know' all that we need to know. And yet we're still missing something…"

The logic behind Newtonian law and its best known principle is that of analysis or reductionism. Newtonian science teaches us that in order to understand any complex phenomenon, you need to take it apart, reduce it to its individual parts. If these are still complex, you need to take your analysis even further, break it down and look at their components.

This is how we do things in the Western medical model, look at an overall system and break it down into parts to treat and cure the problem area. It's become extremely compartmentalized as specific specialties continue to thrive.

This is also similar to what we discussed in chapter two in relation to nursing, problem solving and fixing our difficulties without looking at the root cause, underlying issues or global totality of the concern.

Quantum Physics

Everything is made up of energy. This shouldn't be a very hard sell since all (most?) of you reading this book are nurses.

Think about your body. What is it made up of? The organs and systems that keep us alive. OK, well what are your systems and organs made of? Tissues. Very good. And how about tissues, what are they made up of? (Don't worry; the science test is almost over). Right again! Cells.

Cells are made up of molecules and molecules are made of atoms. Atoms are made of sub-atomic particles, like protons, neutrons and electrons. And what are these made up of?

Energy!

We are pure energy beings as are our material possessions, plants and animals, surrounding environment and even thoughts and feelings. Everything is made up of energy.

Now I am not an expert on quantum physics, nor do I want to bore, confuse or teach you to death but at the very basic level we're living on more than a physical plain. The quantum world proposes that everything we see is merely an illusion of perception. We are all living our own version of reality. What we focus on becomes real and what we don't give attention to just doesn't exist in our world as we know it.

Have you ever experienced an event or situation that wasn't easy? How did everyone in your life respond? I'd bet that no two people had the same reaction. For example, let's say my neighbor's truck was set on fire. He might have responded with a lot of fear, having a hard time adjusting to this traumatic event. On the other hand his wife may have perceived the same situation and reacted with more anger, wanting to get back at whoever vandalized their property. Still further another neighbor, living right next door and witnessing the same event, may have felt gratitude that their house did not catch on fire.

You see what I'm getting at here?

It is all about perception and because of the theories realized through the quantum field we can then understand that energy flows where attention goes.

If all of this is not making sense and confusing you further- don't worry. In the chapters that follow we'll go piece-by-piece into more detail, but we'll use actual tools and techniques that can help you get there. The main aspects you need to understand put simply, are- everything is made of energy. The energy that you put out, via thoughts, feelings, emotions, beliefs and attitudes, vibrates at a certain level and because like attracts like, we want to vibrate at our highest energy levels that we can.

OK. Let's leave the scientific discussion for a moment and come on back to the 'art' of nursing.

What we want to do is bridge the gap between the art and science of nursing, allowing them both to flourish one and the same.

We still need our technical skills, critical thinking and analytical logic. We need to be able to solve problems, put out fires and work in and through fast-paced emergency situations. We need computers, machines and equipment to help us do our jobs efficiently and safely. So how can we do this with a bit of finesse? In what way can we continue to excel at such high-tech roles but thrive in a way that is meaningful and enjoyable for all who are involved?

As the brief introduction into scientific theory is uncovered, it's all about energy. In the next chapter I'm going to cover a spiritual healing practice that intermingles with some energy theories that I've come to learn, know and appreciate on multiple levels.

If you are feeling a bit lost, overwhelmed or confused; don't be. We'll speak more to energy and how this will help us awaken the nurse within in the next chapter and follow that up with actual tools you can use in your daily life to not only survive, but thrive, as a busy, successful and happy nurse.

Elizabeth Scala

5

Experiences in Faith
"The character of a nurse is just as important as the knowledge he/she possesses." -Carolyn Jarvis

I was back at the hospital, working part-time in a clinical nurse research fellowship. My boss knew I was also working part-time at a local gym and really getting into health and wellness. She suggested I head down to the career fair, as there were some holistic modalities set up for sampling.

I put my name down on the long waiting list for acupuncture. I had never had it before and wondered if I would do OK with the needles. I was interested to try it, but one of the women in charge came up to me and said: "You know, there is a long wait for the acupuncturist. Why don't you

34

give the Reiki (*pronounced Ray-key*) a try? No one is doing that right now…"

She handed me a flyer, which I looked over and handed back to her. I didn't even understand what it said. I mean, of course I could read it, but the words I read made no sense to me at all.

Since I had to get back to my office in a shorter time span than the wait for the acupuncture line would allow, I decided to give it a try. "Sure, I'll see the Reiki (*was I even pronouncing it right?*) person," *I timidly whispered.*

I went into the dimly lit room and there was this woman with a big smile on her face. "Come, sit down. What's going on with you?" *I didn't know what to expect; I said something about how I didn't know what Reiki was and mumbled on about how my foot had some pain from the half-marathon I was training for.*

"Sure, sit in this chair. Go ahead and close your eyes. Let the Reiki do the healing."

The entire time I tried to open my eyes and peek. What was she doing? Where was she standing? Was she on my left or my right? How come I felt tingly sensations going down my spine? This is so weird!

After a few moments she was 'done'. "OK. You're all set, let me share a flyer with you. We're holding a class next spring for healthcare professionals who want to learn Reiki. You should join us."

I took the flyer, still had no idea what on earth was going on or had happened, and figured I would never see this woman again. Oh, and that this thing called 'Reiki' wouldn't do a thing for my foot. I mean, she never even touched my foot, so how could it!?!

Boy was I wrong…

That was my introduction to energy, Reiki and the healing power of thought.

Now I had read and watched 'The Secret' a few years before I had the experience I shared above. I understood the 'concepts' and did value what they were saying. It made perfect sense, like the Golden Rule or something, treat others the way you want to be treated.

But this Reiki stuff was way beyond my understanding.

Being a nurse, I'm quite analytical. I enjoyed logic and math during school. I like to understand the reasons behind things and am always listening to the statistical proof. I mean come on, at the time I was working in a research role, right?!

So to tell me that there was this universal life force, this power beyond our control and that it knew where to go to allow for ultimate healing on every level was totally outside of my comfort zone.

To make a long story short, I did take that training in the spring. I still didn't understand what was happening. I only knew that I felt so much better and my foot was fine for the half-marathon I trained for and successfully ran.

So Reiki. What does Reiki have to do with our discussion here? How come we're touching on it now? Where does it fit in relation to trying something new as a nursing profession?

In the previous chapter, with our discussion about the quantum world, we covered the fact that everything is energy. So as I said before, we're made up of energy as is everything around us. Well, there's also a greater source, beyond our own physical being, an energy that is greater than all.

Some call this greater energy 'source' or the 'universe'. Others may attach some sort of God-like qualities to it. In my study and practice of Reiki, I've come to understand it as the life force energy. Reiki, when you break down the two syllables of the word (Rei-ki), literally means 'universal life force energy'.

There is an energy that is greater than ourselves as human beings; there is energy within, around and a part of everything we do, be and are and so our energy can also be our thought.

Why did I tell you the story of how I got introduced to Reiki? Why am I going into such detail on this spiritual healing practice?

Well, I didn't 'get' Reiki. I couldn't understand how it worked; when I really try to sit and think about it (or explain it to the nurses I share it with) I still am not sure I fully understand it. How can this source, this energy beyond me, help me to feel better? How does sitting and practicing Reiki on a daily basis make me feel calmer, happier and more at peace? How does Reiki even work?

I don't know. But what I do know is this: I am experiencing faith.

I am not one hundred percent sure as to what's going on, but I am clear that it is helping. In addition, I was at a point in my life where the 'old way' wasn't working any more. I knew I wanted and needed something different and so I was open to receiving guidance along the way.

Now, let's revisit what I shared with you in terms of the nursing profession.

We've got some age-old issues that continue to resurface and bubble up for us both as a group and as individuals. We keep trying to 'fix' our problems with the same minds that created them. It is now time for a fresh perspective of solutions that will work because these new answers will create empowered nurses who are change agents, happy and healthy with themselves, their lives and each other.

Using quantum physics, energy principles and universal law we know that thoughts influence emotions which in turn, influence actions and behaviors. How can you behave, act and make choices in a new way when you are thinking the same old thing?

It's time to leave the problem-solution based model aside and heal the root cause: the thought.

The old way is putting a band-aid on every little problem as it arises. The way it's 'always been done' is to fix the problem with a solution, but even the best intended solutions create with them unintended side effects. The best way to heal is to get at the root cause, the thought that created them.

Change your thoughts and change your life.

Are you ready to experience faith? Are you open to receiving something new? Are you ready for an epic shift?

This is the time.

It's here.

It's now that you will truly understand and be able to use the power of your mind, your unique sense of self and a conscious choice to uplift your health, self, career and life. Let's get going; the fun's about to begin!

6

Choose Nursing From Within

"I was once asked why I don't participate in anti-war demonstrations. I said that I will never do that, but as soon as you have a pro-peace rally, I'll be there."
—Mother-Teresa

It's a really busy weekend and I'm running charge and acting as NCIII for the floor, which means I round with the weekend attending physician seeing each patient one-by-one. This is all-too common for me, as most shifts I find myself in charge, taking patients of my own, and acting as NCIII for one of our services. It's no different than before- it just has to all get done.

Maybe it's my highly organized nature; maybe it's because I'm a leader in my unit. I'm not exactly sure what it is, but doing both roles at once doesn't faze me too much. Sure, it's not ideal. It's probably not the best thing for my patients or the time I get to spend with them, but we get it done.

When you're in charge on my psych floor you run the community meeting. When you round with the physicians you're seeing patients in the early part of the day. So the team has to help out with my medications and other tasks. Oh yeah, and someone has to cover the phone while I'm in with the doctor.

Yikes! How to do it all?

"Thanks so much for helping me, Eddie," I say when we make it to our morning debriefing huddle. "I'm so grateful you gave those meds out, Katie. Thank you."

I feel really good, knowing I have an awesome team on today. Knowing that my patients are safe and my work is done. Knowing that we are all taking care of each other and working as one.

The day is busy but there is time for laughter. We all get to eat lunch and for that I am forever grateful. We make it out on time and all of the patients received quality care.

Another day is done. Our work was as work goes, but I feel good about it all.

What I described above could sound like a nightmare. Of course, I shared that it all worked out well and I enjoyed my day, but to some of you reading you might be thinking to yourself 'How could you do both roles at once? That isn't safe and/or quality care! I don't understand why you let the staffing get that bad? That day didn't sound good at all to me!'

And you're right.

On the one hand, I didn't see my patients often that day. I didn't have time to sit with them as long as I would have liked. I may have missed a moment where I could have listened, seen or felt.

So maybe I left work with a less meaningful connection than I would have wanted.

OR-

Or I can look at it that we all made it through safe. No one was harmed. The patients were able to get their medications, attend their groups, visit with their families and enjoy a movie. On the weekends, the unit was a bit more relaxed so maybe they didn't need to sit and process and talk and think with me all day long about their problems. Maybe they needed a break!

I've come to create a concept, coin a term if you will, that this entire book is based upon.

Nursing from Within

Sure, nursing is stressful, difficult and tiring work. We've gone through that in the previous chapters of this book. So one perception we could consciously choose to take is to focus on the stress of the job, the challenge of the role.

But guess what?

This stress isn't going anywhere. It's not going away. In fact, I believe it could potentially get even more stressful, much harder, before our nursing climate gets better.

Oh, that sounds bleak. My opinion? It doesn't have to be.

We've got the stress of nursing. It's there. It's real. It's so real it's tangible. OK.

And you've also got a choice.

A choice to know that stress will be there. A choice to flow through and with the stress. A choice of going within, tapping into the reserves and resources that you find inside of yourself. A choice to connect with the spirit of nursing, with the nurse within you.

I opened up this chapter with one of my favorite quotes of all-time. Mother Teresa, in my opinion as evidenced by the words she shared on peace and war, is a true hero. Each and every one of us nurses can learn from her leadership.

And that's just what it is.

I told you in Chapter 3 that it's not always going to be easy, that you might have to stand alone. I shared with you the fact that change may be slow, uncomfortable and difficult. Others may not agree with what you have decided, how you live your life and how you show up being you.

Nursing from within is about being the nurse you want to be. It's about shifting your inner perspective so that you can enjoy your outer environment, no matter how stressful or challenging that may be. Nursing from within is about connecting to your authentic self, your best nurse, and using your skills, talents and abilities to create the experience of your dreams.

You can be a nurse. You can thrive as a nurse. You can work in any nursing environment there is. Even in the worst of situations, even in the most dire circumstances. It's not about the 'job'; it's about how you show up in life. How you perceive your reality. The thoughts that you think which influence the feelings you feel and the actions you take.

To awake the nurse within will require some shifts and that's just what the rest of this book will help you do. In the chapters that follow we will talk about some concepts and strategies that will help you reconnect with the nurse within.

7

Today Only

"The thing that is really hard, and really amazing, is giving up on being perfect and beginning the work of becoming yourself. " –Anna Quindlen

I was driving up to one of my spiritual teacher's houses one humid and rainy spring day. It was the second time I would see him and I wondered what he would have me do today.

Would I be outside again, with my hand on a tree, trying (key word here is try since I don't think I did a very good job) to feel its energy? Would he take me on another drumming journey and have me moving in the middle of the room like an animal (totally felt insane and strange doing that one!)? Would he know what color pants I was wearing as he shared with me the last time that he sent me an energetic message?

What was I getting myself into?!?

I started thinking about the Reiki class I was involved with; I was co-teaching Reiki I and sensing a strange energy in the group.

'Do I impact how people feel? Can I really shift an entire room with my presence? I don't think these women actually are practicing Reiki on themselves. They're all talk and no action. I can't stand when people don't live their talk. It's so fake and it drives me crazy. Oh I can't stand this class at all. What am I doing? I shouldn't even be teaching this...' the thoughts went on and on.

My mind raced the entire drive up to Jeremy's house.

I didn't even realize I was there! 'My, that was a fast drive,' I thought to myself as I pulled into my parking spot. 'I made great time.'

He opens the door and invites me in. We go down to his office.

'How have you been? What have you brought for me today? What would you like to focus on in our session?"

I started in on how I am teaching this class and I don't think I should be and I can't stand the energy and can I really impact people and on and on and on...

"Well, I had an idea to go through the four elements with you" *(he motioned to the candle, water, and piece of wood on the table)* "but, in my opinion, we need to shift gears."

We didn't do anything that day, really. Nothing that he had planned or that I had wanted to learn about. The only thing he shared with me that day was this:

Meditate.

On a daily basis, every morning, in the same fashion and at the same time.

"You're distracted by thought. You're in the past and far out into the future. You're not even aware of your present moment. Are you even listening to me now?"

He was right; I had started to think about my drive to his house again and how I didn't even realize I had made it there when I did.

I was distracted! I wasn't present at all. I don't even think I knew what that was or meant. I don't even think I had any clue of what presence would be.

"I am only going to teach you this meditation if you will do it every single morning, sometime before 7 am."

"Before 7 am!" *I shrieked.* "I don't get out of bed until 7:30. I can't do that. Oh, now I'll have to change around my entire schedule. Oh I don't know if I can do it..."

He cut me off.

Already I was in a tailspin.

"You have to decide right now if you will do it or not. I will only teach you if you will. I believe that you need it, but only you can make that choice…"

I made that choice. That was several years ago. For the first year, almost daily, I got up every morning and did the practice he showed me before 7 am. Since then I've created my own practice, now that I am committed to it.

I did make that choice to learn that day. I knew I needed something. I knew where I was, and it was not where I wanted to be. I knew that I desired something different and I consciously chose to get myself there.

That was several years ago and that meditation practice has made all of the difference.

What Jeremy gifted me with that day was something beyond measure. He empowered me with time. He allowed me to settle. He helped me find comfort, joy and peace of mind in the here-and-now.

How many of you reading this book, right now even, have something else on your mind?

As nurses we struggle with this. We are driving to work and thinking about the day ahead. 'Oh, I hope I don't have to work short-staffed today. I better get out on time. I have to pick up Sara at practice. I really don't want to have a day like we had yesterday…'

It goes on and on.

Or worse: bringing work home with you.

When was the last time you left a shift, worrying if you got everything done? 'Did I hang that bag? Did I tell her about the new medication? Did I call him about that lab value?'

And so on and so on.

We're worrying about things that haven't happened yet or stuck obsessing about things that we have no control over. Did you know that the past is the past and you can't go back in time to fix, edit, or change any of it?

It's over.

In fact, some argue that the past does not even exist.

And we know that the future doesn't exist. It hasn't happened yet. I always let go of a future worry by realizing, hey… I may not even make it that far out! I could die today and not even get to that place where the bill is due.

The only time that really matters, that even exists is right here and right now.

In the appendix of this book, I share with you several resources that have helped me get to the place where I am today with respect to time and the present moment. They will help but reading more information won't actually change a thing.

You actually have to take what you learn and implement it.

That's one of the problems with our culture. We are information addicts. We want more and more knowledge; we learn new skills, take classes, and over inundate ourselves with trainings.

You actually don't need any more information.

What you need is peace and quiet.

You need the present moment.

You need to exist in your here-and-now.

The first line in the Reiki principles is: Just for Today.

Just for today gets you back to the present moment. You know I think about how people set goals and make changes. We say to ourselves, 'OK, this month I am going to start exercising.' Then days come and go and the exercise doesn't happen. But what does happen?

We start to beat ourselves up. We feel guilty for the fact we never get started. We think we're a failure and say 'Oh here I go again, another goal I didn't reach.'

Guess what?

You've over-extending yourself. You set yourself up for failure. Living in the future or the past is a form of self-sabotage. The only way to truly reach a goal and have success is to make a conscious choice in that present moment.

In that moment you can choose to stay on the couch, in front of the TV, or you can choose to get up and go for a walk. Exercise. Or not.

'Just for today' is a statement of empowerment.

Now, let's relate all of this back to nursing, our roles as busy nurses and our desire to connect with our nurse within.

Picture a busy scene in your workplace. You're rushing from here-to-there. This person needs this while another person on the phone needs that and neither of those people are your patient who needs to get prepped for their procedure.

How will you handle it all? How can you get thirty things done at once?

It may be difficult and you may want to slap me. In fact, you probably won't even believe it can happen. Remember, these shifts take practice, time and faith.

How can you do it? The answer: Stay present to the moment you are in.

Breathe, exhale and say to yourself: "Just for today."

The more you can stay present in a busy moment the happier you will feel. You will enjoy your job and, in fact, you'll be able to get *more* done with less.

I know. It's sounds crazy. But it's very, very true.

Without distraction, without the future focus or preoccupation with the past, you will enjoy greater productivity, efficiency and peace of mind.

You will. Trust me, I know from experience and practice.

Yup, there's the key word. Practice. It takes practice and again you must implement. It's not just about me writing these words here, you reading them now and thinking to yourself, 'OK- be present'. It's not even just about reading the books I recommend in the back of this book. It's not about tapes, CDs, lectures or workshops.

It's about actually doing it.

Practicing.

So, how do you practice being present in the moment? With some sort of mindfulness practice or meditation on a daily basis.

The only way you will get good at presence in action is practicing presence outside of action.

I sit on my purple block on a daily basis. In absolute quiet. Yes, it's hard. Some days I sit there thinking to myself, 'This isn't working. Oh drat! I'm thinking again. How is this 'right' when I'm distracted right now!?!'

That isn't the point.

There is no right or wrong with sitting in silence, being present to the moment.

Thoughts will come and they will take over. Your job is to notice that, come back to your present moment and let them go.

Over and over and over again.

Practice presence in the quiet to enjoy it in the chaos.

Go within to shift without.

Remember, nursing from within is about making inner shifts so that you can more fully enjoy your external environment. Here is the first tool to start you on your way.

Practice presence and invite it in the here-and-now.

8

Stand Into Your Power

"What you resist, persists." –Carl Jung

'Don't worry about it; I'll come pick you up,*" my husband says over the phone. I'm at work and it's been snowing all afternoon, which wouldn't be an issue but the challenge is I biked to work today.*

'Nah, I'm fine. The roads aren't really even covered yet. I can make it home real quick. I'd rather not leave my bike here, anyway.*"*

'No. I'm coming to get you. That's that. No further discussion,*" Drew states with conviction.*

'How strange,' I'm thinking as I walk to the staff office to clock out. 'Why is he putting up such a big stink?' as I walk my bike inside to the garage.

In the next moment, I get my answer. And my entire universe shifts.

"Your uncle is dead. He's hung himself today. Eddie found him. Please call me," *my mother's sobbing voice stings through the phone.*

I feel like I've just been shot. A drenching wave of vomit, tears and confusion is instantaneously my life.

There's my husband with the car. I'm standing on the corner, sobbing hysterically and getting into the vehicle. Now I know why he wanted to pick me up.

"I wanted to tell you," *he says through his own tears.*

I've never seen Drew this upset before.

We walk into the house; my bags are packed and at the door. "We're leaving tonight. I've taken care of everything. We're staying at your sisters in Brooklyn and we'll be at your uncles first thing in the morning."

I feel such love and support, thank goodness, as it's completely mixed in with sheer shock.

I go upstairs to make some calls. I can't go to work, so I need to tell my two bosses what has happened. I find myself on the phone with a friend.

"I'm almost relieved," *I whisper. As soon as I say it, I'm completely furious.*

'How can I think that about my uncle? Don't I love him deeply? He's gone. Forever. And you're saying you're relieved? What's wrong with you??'

The guilt is palpable.

"No. Not relieved. This is insane. I can't believe this. Is this happening? How terrible. Oh my gosh." *I don't even know how to talk about it.*

I sit at the kitchen table, putting a few forkfuls of spaghetti into my mouth. I can't chew. I can't taste. The feelings are different on a moment-by-moment basis.

Shock. Fear. Sadness. Anger. Disbelief. What the Hell is going on!?

And time passes on. Day by day. It's been over three years since the day I received that call. I'm still here. And so is my family. Life happens on…

Wow.

What an event. To relive that story, to retell those events- I can feel those physical feelings right now in this moment as I type these words.

My heart racing, the nausea, and the tears- it is all here. Right now. As if it's happening again today.

Feelings of anger, frustration and confusion towards my uncle. Why did you do it? How could you do it? Emotions of sadness, disbelief and loss. My family! Going through something like this? How can that be?

And as I said- it's been more than three years since the day it happened. More than 36 months. More than 1,000 days.

What's happened to me is what happens to us all.

When we relive an experience we don't only think of the events or speak words to the situations. When a memory has that much emotion all tangled up with it; we are physically, emotionally and mentally living that very day, all over again.

It's as if he's dying right now. It's as though my mother has left me that voice mail message. It's like my father is standing in our living room telling his wife that her youngest brother has hung himself.

It's happening again.

And it's unhealthy for all of us. To relive the events that have happened, those things that we can never change or figure out why. To continuously play the tape over and over in our minds, bringing up these negative emotions, does more harm than good.

I am sharing this with you as an example. This story is one that is completely extreme and I chose it on purpose. I needed an event that conjured up emotions, felt deep within. I am telling you this to teach our next lesson here as we journey together upon connecting with the nurse within.

It is time to let go.

Let go of the guilt, blame, shame, fear, doubt, worry, criticism and darkness. Let go of the pain, sadness, anger, resentment and jealousy. Let go of negative thoughts, emotions, feelings, behaviors and actions.

Let go.

Now letting go may not always be easy. In fact, it might be very difficult. I was once asked by one of my Reiki I students, *"Elizabeth, I understand the concept in words but I can't seem to release the anger I feel. How do I do this?"*

Such a great question. Maybe a question that doesn't even have a one-size fits all response.

I heard a great speaker talk to this very idea of forgiveness. The teaching point was that while we may never forget that memory of hurt done to us, what's the point of holding onto the feeling of the pain?

Holding onto tension, pain, stress and fear actually harms us as we attempt to harm the individual that hurt us. Our holding onto these negative emotions creates blockage, inflammation and actual harm to the physical body.

Letting go allows energy to flow. It allows movement. It invites shifts. Letting go can free us from the pain.

Sharing the story of the day I received the news that my uncle had passed away, highlights how strong, deep and intertwined the emotions can be. It's a hard memory to conjure up. And it's getting easier every time I do.

Why?

Because I am letting go.

I have let go of the guilt for not being more aware of the pain that he was in. I've let go of the anger I had towards him for choosing to leave the physical plain. I've let go of some sadness as I am mindful of his smile, laugh and joy every time I look in the mirror and smile at my own self. I've let go and continue to let go each and every day. I forgive myself and my uncle and move forward.

So let's relate this back to you, to your work as a nurse, and to our connection to nursing from within.

What mistakes have you made at work that you're still beating yourself up over? Which tragic patient memories are hard to shake? What colleague, manager or even institution are you still feeling hurt or disrespected by? What are you still holding on to? And are you ready to forgive?

There's a wonderful little tale I learned in my Reiki education. It goes something like this...

Two monks are walking the bank of a river one day and they see a woman drowning in the water beside them. Although it's against their custom to engage in physical contact with the opposite sex, one of the monks reaches in and helps the woman out to safety.

Time passes and almost a half of an hour later, the monk that rescued the woman looks to his friend and asks, *"Why are you so silent? What is angering you?"*

"You picked that woman up! It's against everything we believe in."

"Why dear friend," the monk smiles in response, *"You're the one still carrying that woman upon your back. I let her down several miles back. It's you that cannot let her go..."*

When we hold onto things they become heavy. We are literally weighted down by our own emotions and feelings. The energy is stuck, thick and gooey, like glue.

Yes, it may be very hard to let go of something so painful. Something that induces such strong anger, despair and/or fear, but what good is it doing holding onto it? Who is it serving?

You might say it's a way we protect ourselves.

"I hold onto that anger so that I don't let myself get hurt again."

"I keep up that fear so that I don't look foolish in the future."

These are protective mechanisms, but who are they protecting really? The only thing these holds are doing is keeping us small and dark.

The Marianne Williamson quote can sum this point up the best. She says:

"Our deepest fear is not that we are inadequate. Our deepest fear is that we are powerful beyond measure. It is our light, not our darkness that most frightens us. We ask ourselves, 'Who am I to be brilliant, gorgeous, talented, and fabulous?' Actually, who are you not to be? You are a child of God. You're playing small does not serve the world. There is nothing enlightened about shrinking so that other people won't feel insecure around you. We are all meant to shine, as children do. We were born to make manifest the glory of God that is within us. It's not just in some of us; it's in everyone.

And as we let our own light shine, we unconsciously give other people permission to do the same. As we are liberated from our own fear, our presence automatically liberates others."

Let's take this conversation back to our nursing practice.

Where are you playing small? How might you be holding back? What can you release to allow the nurse inside of you to shine?

I would like to share an exercise that I do on a daily basis that has helped me in letting go. I hope this practice serves you in some way. Again, this is a practice. It is something that the more you choose to do it, the more benefit will come. So let's get to it.

I am sure you've heard of affirmations before. They're all over the self-help world. And for a while I was so frustrated by affirmations, thinking that they just don't work!

I even taught that for a while: affirmations don't work and here's why.

Well, in one way I was right. But on the flip side I was totally wrong. Let's talk a bit about affirmations and then I'll share my practice with you.

Affirmations are statements that you may say to yourself or aloud, with the intent to change something about yourself. You want more of something or you'd like to let something go. So, you create a statement, repeat it over and over and then hope for the shift.

This is the way that most people do affirmations and, unfortunately, the way they're usually taught.

This is why the affirmations aren't producing the shifts you are looking for. You haven't gotten to the root cause of the concern at hand. Just like in chapter two when we discussed how band-aids don't fix things, this concept surfaces here.

So what's the trouble? In addition to the fact that we're not getting at the underlying issues many of us are lining up our affirmations all wrong.

In the past, you may have tried an affirmation that used negative language, saying something like "I don't want to worry any more" and what you may or may not have noticed, was that in stating an affirmation in this way, you actually get more worry than less of it. You see, the universe doesn't comprehend the word 'not'. Stating an affirmation such as "*I don't want to worry anymore*" actually is like saying "*I'd like to continue with my worry*".

Also, you may not have truly and completely believed in your actual power to have the affirmation come true, thus setting yourself up for total failure. Saying something like, "*I'd like to have more money*" but not really believing that more money can come to you creates that very manifestation of not having money again.

You see, we have our conscious mind and our subconscious mind. The conscious mind can say one thing, but if the subconscious mind isn't on board, no progress will evolve.

We've got to invite ourselves to the possibility of the shift we are intending to bring about. The language we use is very specific and doing it in this way creates those affirmations that actually do work.

It's all in use of one small word. Want to know what that word is?

Choose

Instead of:

I believe it's easy for me to be self-confident.

It would be:

I choose to believe it's easy for me to be self-confident.

How does that sound? Better yet, how does it feel? Pretty different, right? It's much more believable when we invite the choice into it. Because then, over time, what's happening is, we are allowing our subconscious mind to get on board with the shift.

Instead of shocking it into something totally new and foreign to our being, we are gently inviting more of what we want into our lives. If you've never been self-confident before and you're standing there affirming that you want to be, you're going to have a very hard time convincing the subconscious mind that you can do it. You've got all of this past experience behind you, showing you otherwise.

Yet if you invite it in, slowly over time, you will enjoy remarkable results.

Trust me. I know from experience.

Remember how I told you that I didn't believe that affirmations worked? I wasn't seeing results. Well introducing the word 'choose' into my intentional affirmations I've created some actual shifts and am enjoying the beneficial consequences of my practice.

Here's an actual example for you.

I have had some major history with rejection. Growing up, I encountered multiple betrayals from people very close to me. Boys wouldn't even talk to me in high school and my 'best' friends completely disowned me. These experiences made it very hard for me to approach anyone about anything at all.

I always felt I would be told 'no'.

So, I used to say affirmations about creating more confidence. I used unclear language without much intention. On a subconscious level, I probably also doubted it would even work.

Then, I learned about using the word 'choose'. On a daily basis I've looked in the mirror, smiling at myself in a genuine way, and said: I choose to make it easy for me to be self-confident.

You know what's happened to me recently?

I've actually been able to pick up the telephone and call complete strangers, offering my speaking, teaching and presenting services to their nursing groups. Wow! What a major shift.

What a way that I am stepping into my light, allowing my greatness to shine. What an example of letting go of the fear, doubt and worry of what may happen when I pick up the phone.

This brings us back to letting go.

What is it that you'd like to let go of with respect to your nursing career? What would you like to have more of? How can you use the practice of intentional affirmations to release the old and invite the new?

It surely is a practice and it most likely will take time, but it's so worth it.

When you strip away the unnecessary layers of your small self, you will find an amazing treasure inside. Letting go allows you to get closer and closer to the nurse within. In the next chapter we will welcome a beautiful practice that will wonderfully complement our work we've just completed. So let's journey on.

9

The Pleasure of Practice

"The way we communicate with others and with ourselves ultimately determines the quality of our lives." -Anthony Robbins

When I moved to the home that I live in today, it was an extreme change for me. The 2 mile distance from my work to my home the past decade was over. I could no longer bike to work; rather I'd find myself in a one-hour commute, each way.

Yes, I had wanted the country life. I longed for my own grass, trees and outside living space. I wanted distance between myself and my neighbors. I longed for peace and quiet.

Now, I found myself sitting in the car, something I vowed I would never waste my time doing in my adult life. I wasn't one of 'those' people, miserably shuffling back and forth to work.

Turns out, I'm not one of those people.

The car has become an interesting place for me. Not only do I get some serious chair-dancing time in, but I've been able to really heal, grow and change. I took up some universal law course work and the neat thing was a lot of it was done via mp3 audio.

Yup, so I got to download this to my iPod and pop it into the car ride to and from my hospital job.

Another blessing I've come across in my zippy blue Honda CRZ is the inspiration, awe and feeling of total connection. Nature is a beautiful thing.

Some mornings I am blessed with watching the sun rise as I wind up over another hill. Other days, I am able to catch an entire flock of small black birds, landing in unison across the cornfields. Last winter we had this incredible ice storm that, while it left us without power for some time, the way that the trees sparkled and danced in the sunlight was beyond breathtaking.

Even as I sit here, typing these words and reliving these gifts from Mother Nature, tears are forming in my eyes.

What beauty. A feeling of pure love. Complete and total support. Trust in the fact that this is a beautiful and loving world and I'm so lucky to be a part of it today.

In previous chapters we've touched on how hard nursing work can be and I don't think I even mentioned the shift work. We go in at all hours of the day and work all hours of the night.

Traveling to-and-from work, back and forth, come and go. It can become quite mundane. In fact, I've heard of a nursing shuffle. It's that hustle, head down as you walk robotically into your next shift.

It isn't pretty.

Another common challenge in the commute is the actual travel itself and our use of time. Do you listen to the morning news, filled with scarcity and fear? Do you think about your day ahead, worrying about who you might be working with or what colleague may not show up?

The time to-and-from work can be a curse or a blessing in disguise.

I opt for the latter.

In fact, I opt for the latter in every single situation and experience we encounter.

The third concept that will invite a reconnection with the nurse within is allowing yourself to find the joy, appreciation and gratitude in it all.

Since our previous chapter was all about letting go, when we release the negative we open up the flow. We make space. What is it you want to make space for?

Something beautifully magnificent, I hope!

Now I know some of you reading may be conjuring up some objections here. 'This sounds too Polly-Anna for me,' your inner critic may oppose.

Yes, I'm certainly aware of life and the ups-and-downs that can occur, but guess what? There's an opportunity here for empowerment. A chance to totally tip the scales in your favor. A way to decrease the 'downs' and revel in longer joy of the 'ups'.

A golden nugget from some passage I read a long time ago, one that I've never forgotten and still use daily to this day, is this:

Every situation is an opportunity for learning, growth, healing and change.

Every situation.

It's a gift. Each moment is a chance to learn something new; an opportunity to make a conscious choice. A way for you to grow through something and thrive on the other side.

You may even choose to play around with the wording and invite the statement into your daily intentional affirmation practice:

71

I choose to view every situation as an opportunity for learning, growth, healing and change.

Wow. How powerful is that?

OK, so besides this notion that we can learn and grow from every situation, what about appreciation, joy and gratitude?

Oh! The opportunities are endless.

As you move throughout your nursing shift, what can you be grateful for? As you interact with people during your day, what can you appreciate in each one of them? As you take a moment to pause in the present moment what joy is occurring, right now?

The possibilities are infinite.

In previous chapters we covered energy, emotion, thought and how what we focus on we get more of. Choosing to give your attention to the joy, appreciation and gratitude as you interact with the experiences of your day only brings you more of the same.

Another common protest that arises when we speak of looking for the positive in all things is this: what about other people? She's so nasty; he's such a worry-wart. How do I interact with the world and still find the good in it all?

Yes. The world is out there and people will be as they choose to be. That's the gift. We all have a choice. On top of that choice is also being grounded in reality. You can never, ever know what another person is thinking, feeling or going to do. You can influence them, but you can't change them. Role-modeling, mentoring or showing the way through our actions may lead to changes in others, but ultimately it is up to them.

As I shared in Chapter Eight, the end of Marianne Williamson's quote says this best:

"And as we let our own light shine, we unconsciously give other people permission to do the same. As we are liberated from our own fear, our presence automatically liberates others."

When you make the conscious choice to look for the good, revel in the joy, engage in appreciation and find space for gratitude- just your very actions- will inspire others to do the same. They will see how you show up; they will feel your energy. They will want some of what you've got going on and they'll start to shift in the same way.

So, a practice I'd like to introduce and share with you here is one of giving thanks. Expressing gratitude on a daily basis and feeling it.

I'm sure you've heard of gratitude before. Lately it's become a very popular idea. With gratitude journals, morning gratitude exercises and lots of self-help gurus talking about the power of gratitude, expressing thanks has taken center stage.

In most cases, I choose to steer clear of the crowd, but in terms of gratitude- all of these people telling you to practice it- they are right. Often, what's missing are two crucial caveats that I will cover with you right now.

First off, gratitude is best practiced EVERYDAY. You must. As simple as brushing your teeth or going to the bathroom, you do these things every single day, right? Gratitude is the same thing. You can't do it one day and expect for everything to change.

So you've got to practice gratitude on a daily basis. The more you can be thankful for, every single day, the more things to be thankful for will come.

The other piece to this, which not many people talk about, is feeling it. It's more than simply expressing the gratitude in words. I did this for a while.

I saw the movie 'The Secret' and I was like, 'Oh I get it'. I 'understood' the concept in theory. I could recite back to you what the Law of Attraction was saying. But did I live it? Initially, no.

It was a lot of parroting back what I read and heard, grasping it in my mind, but not in my heart. Stating the information instead of living the skill. As nurses we are sort of at risk here.

We can learn clinical skills, watching an instructor teach us what it is we are to do. We may even pass an exam, mentally grasping the information. But unless we actually do it, use it in our practice; are we living the new skill in our lives? Are we incorporating these skills into our work routines?

As a psychiatric nurse, I lacked many of the 'medical' nursing-type skills. I can remember we had a patient on our floor that had a tracheotomy. My oh my, were we scared!

No one wanted to have this patient. During the day it wasn't that bad because the medical nurse would come by and see him. But at night, when we were all alone, just two of us, it was always a fear that I'd have to perform this task.

I understood what I was supposed to do. I watched someone else do it. I read about it. I could tell you how to do it properly. I even knew what equipment to use and what safety precautions were needed. But to actually do it without embedding that experience into my life; I was terrified.

The same holds true with gratitude (well, maybe not the fear piece).

You can understand the concept; you can even say 'I'm thankful for' in words. But, unless you put meaning and feeling behind the actual prose; you won't get the most bang for your buck.

Attaching a feeling to it is so much more powerful.

Why?

Emotions are powerful clues. In addition, emotions are attached to thoughts. Feelings get stored in our psyche.

It's not 'Oh, I remember when I got lost as a little girl'. It's the feeling of being lost that you remember. The terror that your parents would never find you. The confusion that was overwhelming. The tears that gushed as you got more and more stressed out. You feel that memory; you don't just 'say' it.

When you practice your daily gratitude, you must attach an emotion to it. Why does the person, place or thing that you are expressing gratitude for make you feel good? What feeling comes from that situation, event or idea that you are thankful for?

Instead of *'I'm thankful for my family'* it's *'I'm thankful for my dogs because they make me feel silly, playful and full of cheer'*. Then as you say it, feel those feelings.

I take it as far as saying my gratitude list while looking in the mirror. I smile at myself and really feel the joy coming from inside of my heart. It's something I've committed to doing on a daily basis.

As I shared in my vignette about my daily commute to work, I'm certainly enjoying the results… and so can you!

10

Go for Your Dreams

"To accomplish great things, you must not only act, but also dream, not only plan, but also believe." -Anatole France

It was late summer and I was getting ready to graduate from my Masters' programs that December. I'd have a degree in business and nursing and knew I wanted to do something different with it.

I was standing on my front porch of my parents' beach house in Cape May, New Jersey. On the other end of the phone was my academic advisor, a very experienced nurse with lots of background in various roles and capacities. People knew her name and she was well-respected in the profession. I was so glad and grateful this was my academic advisor.

"I want to do something with prevention in mind. I know I like to plan and organize so something where I might be strategically planning, maybe teaching something about prevention. I'm not really sure. I just know I want to be involved with preventing people from needing to go to a hospital. What can I do? Any ideas?"

Kathi was very wise, helpful and kind in her responses to me. She suggested some possibilities, directed me to other people who I might talk to for more information. She even offered some places I might look at for jobs like I was describing.

I continued on throughout the rest of the summer, telling everyone and anyone that would listen what I wanted to do with my life.

"I just want to work in prevention. I want to help people stay well. "

Over and over again I'd say what I wanted, not really being exactly clear on what that would look like or how that might play out.

I went on some job interviews, never really landing any of the roles, and I continued forward. "I just want to help with well-being, wellness. "

Fall came and I was in my final course of the dual degree program, a practicum that was all-inclusive as a means to capture and bring together everything that we had learned over the past few years. I had chosen to do my capstone project through the student exchange program that the university had all set up with colleagues in Germany.

The German students came for a week in October and our group gathered working daily on our final deliverable. Our charge: go into a health club in the area and research, review and recommend a marketing plan for their up-and-coming social media campaign.

A health club! What an awesome opportunity. I'd be around wellness all week.

Well, this actually turned out to be more than a simple coincidence; this would be my new career. A woman on the project said to me, "You're a nurse and you're going to have your masters' degree. You're just what we're looking for to head-up a new program at our downtown location."

Music to my ears.

So, I became the Healthy Start Nurse for an elite wellness center in Baltimore, Maryland. What sticks out so vividly in my mind was that phone call with Kathi, my advisor, at the beach. "I want to be in prevention. I want to coordinate, strategize, teach and plan. I'm not sure what it is; I just want to be in wellness…"

This next chapter is extremely important for our goal with connecting with nursing from within. It's all about what's inside us. Becoming and being our highest expression of our authentic selves.

Before I get ahead of myself though, there are a few pieces of the puzzle that I must absolutely touch on. A laying of the foundational framework, so to speak.

As adults, we are at a disadvantage. Since we've had to 'grow up' and navigate the world that we live in, many of us have lost touch with our sense of self. We think with our heads instead of our hearts. Being disconnected from the heart is an extreme disservice as we go forward through this chapter's material.

So, before we get into anything new I invite you to open up to a new way. Or as some may see it, an 'old' way as this was the way we did things as children do. This heart-based connection is something all of us had, some time before our present day.

If I were to ask you what you wanted, many of you would start to 'think' about it. "*Hmm*," you might say, "*What is it I want...*" Then you'd probably get all wrapped up in the amount of resources, time, energy or money it would take to get what you wanted, which could potentially sabotage you before you even got started.

I'm not talking about what you 'think' you want here in this book. It isn't an exercise for the head.

What I'm describing here is very different. Instead of 'thinking' about what you want, I encourage you to feel for what you want. What is it that your true heart desires?

Opening up to your true hearts desires is a key to lifelong success.

See what happens is this: when you think about what you want your limited mind, based on your past experiences, memories, perceptions, beliefs, education and upbringing, creates a picture of what it thinks you 'should' want. What's possible for you based on what you know.

Even further, what your mind wants usually isn't what your true self, that highest expression of your authentic you, really desires. Tapping into the heart's desires, on the other hand, aligns you with what you truly long for.

That is why so many of us fail at setting goals. We haven't taken the time to stop and feel what it is we truly are after. We set a goal based on what other people have done, what we've seen work for that group over there, what someone else has told us we'd be good at doing, or other exterior influences that really are meaningless when it comes to the heart.

The heart is your connection to your highest self, the connection to your soul. The heart never lies. Your heart, what you truly and deeply desire deep inside, can go after and therefore achieve whatever it wants. When you're traveling the path of the true heart's desires, you won't need motivation or will power to see you through. You will succeed purely because this is what the heart wants.

And what the heart wants, the heart gets.

OK. So I hope you're beginning to see just how important going after what your heart desires really is.

The next step in the foundational framework is taking a powerful pause to get really clear on what it is you want.

How can a contractor build a home without a blueprint? How can you get to your vacation destination without a road map or GPS? You've got to chart a clear path, knowing the course you are going to take to get to A from B.

Many of us want to jump right into action. I see this all the time when people start talking about setting and reaching goals. 'If I want to lose weight I've got to start exercising.' Then, they jump into action without any real pause to consider if this is even the action that's right for them.

Doing the pre-work of figuring out your heart's desires will help you with this. You'll have much more clarity and going after what your heart truly wants will help you take a much more inspired action.

Reconnecting to the nurse within is about knowing what *you* want, for a change, and going for it. Being able to provide nursing care *on purpose* invites you to feel the heart in healing again.

Nursing these days has over-complicated itself. We have certifications for everything. We're required to do training all over the place. We're adding letters upon letters upon letters after our names.

What does it all mean?

Well, if you're not happy with nursing anymore, it quite literally means nothing at all. No letter, fancy title or extra certification, training or degree is going to help you enjoy your career again. It's not more information that you need.

It's about getting back to your nursing desires, your true heart's desires, which come from within.

So, I'm not a huge fan of 'steps' since those models seem very cookie-cutter to me. Yet in this case I think it makes perfect sense to outline for you here the 6 very simple steps that this process can take.

1. Figure out your true hearts desires.

2. Go after what you want, instead of away from what you don't want.

3. Have a clear vision of where you are going.

4. Feel how it will be when that vision comes to fruition.

5. Be open to opportunities, insights, resources and synchronicities.

6. Have fun.

Pretty simple, right?

There's no need to overcomplicate this. The process does work. We've covered the hearts desires and going after what you want quite a bit now, so let's move on to the visioning piece and finish up with the fun.

Vision work is actually very useful. We see in pictures. We think in emotions. We attach feeling to the words that we use.

Once you get clear on what it is you want, there's no need to worry about 'how' you will get there. (This has been one of my most difficult lessons to learn; so trust me on this one. I know from experience that the 'how' may totally surprise you!).

When you have a vision of what you want your ideal nursing role to look and feel like, surround yourself with that vision of you at your best. You can write about this vision; you may sit on a meditation block and see it in your mind's eye. You may want to create a vision board, gathering clippings of images, words and things that instill that vision inside of you.

Whatever it is, however you do it, you simply want to be sure you have that vision in front of you and you are feeling into it on a daily basis.

This is another exercise that will take some conscious practice. It won't work as well to just think about the vision one day, create a vision board and then do nothing with it. You've got to consistently bring that vision to life, to feeling, and allow yourself to imagine what it will be like when you are living and breathing that vision in reality.

Step 5 above goes along with what I've just mentioned about being open to the 'how' of your desires. Sometimes the universal plan and our highest expression of self has a better idea of how we might get from A to B. Choosing to be open to guidance and support brings a level of trust and connection that is so comforting. It allows things to flow much easier, instead of our often-futile attempts at forced action.

The final part of this process is my absolute favorite. Maybe it's because it's one of my own hearts desires.

Fun.

I love talking about the fun.

Richard Simmons once said: "If it ain't fun; it ain't gonna get done."

The nurse within you is alive and well. You just have to tap into him/her, allow her/him to be. This is where the passion for practice comes into play.

If you've found yourself empty, lacking enthusiasm, for the work that you do it may be time to take a good, hard look at your role.

'Work' doesn't have to feel like 'work'. There are people going to work on a daily basis, feeling as if it is play. What a vision, right!?! Here's another that might blow your mind: would you do your job if you weren't even getting paid for it?

That's the space we want to get to with respect to our nursing careers.

We're gifted with such a profound opportunity on a daily basis. We help people heal. We care for those in need. We advocate for the powerless. We give a voice to the weak. We're helpers, teachers, care-givers and friends.

Can you bring more play into your role? Can you have fun with your career? What will it take for you to enjoy your job again?

Nursing from within is about finding your passions, your purpose and working with integrity on a daily basis. Nursing from within is about enjoying your job so it doesn't have to feel like work anymore.

11

Love Turned Inward Ripples Out

"The most powerful relationship you will ever have is the relationship with yourself." –Steve Maraboli

I made the decision to leave my job and go work at the wellness center. Now I come from a family, as many of us my age do, where my parents have been in the same role (one who's been at the same company) their entire lives.

It's just how people of older generations were/are. They get a job, hold the job and keep that job. Until they retire.

Many of us today now know that those days are becoming obsolete. But if you have parents with that mindset, you might feel a little nervous about bringing up the 'I'm leaving my job' topic with them.

I danced around it some, telling them how unhealthy I was feeling. I even shared with them my school project and the words of the employees at the wellness center, how they were looking for a Registered Nurse to run an entire program.

I mean, running a program that had to sound good- right?

Wrong.

Any time I brought up even the notion of leaving my job things like financials, job security, benefits, and perks were all pressed upon me as sparkling jewels and fancy reasons of why I could never leave my hospital job.

One day, I did it.

I put in my letter of resignation; I worked my last shifts. I was out of there. Starting my new job was fun and exciting.

Oh yes, and one day I did this too. "Hi, there," I said to the answering machine in a rushed sort of way, "Yes, everything's coming along nicely here. We're recovering from the two back-to-back blizzards well… Oh yeah and by the way, I quit my job, gotta run… Bye!" *Click.*

I can't remember the repercussions of my decision. I mean, let's face it, I'm still here, alive to tell the story about it today. So, it must not have been that bad, right Dad? LOL.

So yes, I did it. I left my safe and secure, highly paid, well-benefited job to go work part-time at some wellness center. With no benefits, no PTO, nothing, and about a third of the salary.

Was I nuts?

Not at all.

It wasn't about the money anymore, as I come to learn it never really is.

It was about self.

And more than sense of self. Choosing self. Finding self. Allowing self. Loving self.

And that's that. One word. A short, simple word. A challenging concept.

Love.

You know the stories I tell, the ones in this book and the others in my workshops, retreats and talks, may make it sound like things were very bleak. However, this isn't the case at all and was never my intention.

My life is wonderful. Growing up, we had everything we needed, wanted and more. I've taken fascinating trips and enjoyed sports, dance classes, Girl Scouts and fun. I'm totally blessed here and now. My life is full of prosperous abundance.

Many of you reading may resonate and feel the same way. What I find so fascinating though is this: when did I lose the feeling of self-love? How did it go missing along the way?

Because that's what it really all boils down to.

When you strip away the stress, what's beneath the stress, layer upon layer of the onion peel, you get to a simple fact. Simple, but challenging in its reality.

Self-love.

Is it all but gone away?

How many of us are able to tell our parents that we love them? How many times a day do you think about the love that you have for your child? Even those furry friends that greet us when we return from a long, hard shift- don't you love them too?

We are able to send 'I love you' cards for holidays, buy gifts for our lovers and spouses, send flower, chocolates and trinkets to celebrate another person in our life- but what about us? When was the last time you sent yourself an 'I love you' card?

Do you love you?

Really and truly. Unconditionally love you?

Love without judgment. Love without criticism. Love without 'when I look pretty'. Do you love yourself inside and out? Love the good, bad and the ugly? Love every cell of your being? Love the parts of you that are sick or in pain? Do you love your mind, your emotions, your spirit?

Love can be hard.

I won't sit here and pretend I have all of the answers to self-love. But I can tell you this. I've worked on self-love and to be able to make the difficult decisions that I've made in my life; I love me today.

Awhile back, I did some research, interviewing a lot of nurse entrepreneurs on an inquiry that kept replaying itself over and over in my mind.

"Why do you think nurses have such a hard time taking care of themselves?"

I'd ask and listen and we'd talk and discuss.

You see, during the years I had put on several nursing conferences over the virtual space. Hundreds of nurses would sign up, so jazzed about the event and then we'd actually get to the live calls and a handful of people would show. Not only that, in many of the discussion groups of these webinars we'd actually dive into why we as nurses know this self-care stuff but don't actually do it well.

"I'm not a priority," I'd hear. *"I don't have time,"* they'd say.

'OK, so how come you're not a priority? What's underneath that?' My need to get at the underlying root-cause would ponder.

A theme emerged that I thought I'd one day write about, but have never done. Could it be that we, as nurses, have become addicted to taking care of others?

In the interviews I did I heard about nurses burning bridges with family members, nurses in denial that they even had an issue with their health, nurses turning to a healthy solution only when tragedy struck: all very similar concepts to what addicts struggle with in the throes of their addiction.

Now I'm not even sure this is making any sense at all and as of lately I've had a different view of addictions altogether. But, what I am saying, what I believe, is that there is something underneath the 'not taking care of self' that is frequently experienced by the busy nurse.

There's something beneath that and beneath that and that and that and that… Layers upon layers can be peeled away and what I've come to notice is it's all wrapped up in love.

Being too busy, over inundated with information, being plugged in all of the time, rushing from here to there and taking care of others. Not taking care of self. Overdoing it, overcompensating, overexerting.

Where's the love?

It's outward.

The love is expressed all over the place. It's to them. It's for them. I share it with them. I do it here and there and everywhere but the place that it matters most.

Self-Love.

To reconnect with the nurse within means that you love this person that you are. Just as you are. Loving you as you. Being you and no one else. Loving yourself.

So how can we do this? Because I'm well aware that even reading the words in this very chapter may be somewhat uncomfortable for some of you out there. And that's OK. It's totally normal. There's nothing wrong with you.

Self-Love is not something we teach; it isn't something we talk about. And it's certainly something that gets lost along the way.

I'll share with you my practice and invite you to try it too. If it resonates and works for you, great. If not, I encourage you, if you do nothing else after reading this book- at the very least- find a practice of self-love that lands for you.

OK, here we go.

For me, it's smiling inside and out.

As I shared in Chapter Eight, I love my smile. I really do. It's large. It's toothy. It's wide and open. It reminds me of my family members, as we share the same smiles.

I just love how it makes me feel. I love how when I smile at a stranger, they smile back after seeing my huge grin. I love smiling when I laugh. I smile over the phone and on radio interviews and I constantly receive feedback: "Oh, I can hear your smile through the line."

It warms my heart.

I was once working with a coach named Coach Betty Louise. She's all about helping her clients really feel into their bodies, which is difficult because my past and upbringing was more of a cerebral nature. I used to be 'in my head' a lot. So getting into my body when I was coaching with her was a challenge for me.

Well, on one call I believe Coach Betty realized this and said: "Can you feel yourself smiling right now?"

Of course I could.

"Elizabeth, I want you to try to move that smile inside of your body. Can you work on feeling that smile going down into your heart, into your belly and expanding into your entire body until it reaches every cell?"

This I could understand. This I could do. "Yes!" I exclaimed with surprise and glee, "Coach Betty, Yes! I can do this!"

We were both more than thrilled.

Now I had a practice that I could feel into and it was my smile.

Well since then, I've evolved this practice even further. It's meshed into my self-love practice. I smile inside and out, my whole body smile, at least once per day.

When I feel the smile and move it through my body, reaching every single cell, I am bathing myself in loving joy.

I love myself.

Just as I am. As I am meant to be. All of me. Strengths, challenges. Mind, body, spirit. Inside and out. I love me as I am.

And I take this practice now one step further.

When I do the intentional affirmations, my daily gratitude's and the other spiritual practices I've shared along the way in this book, I do it with my smile.

Now maybe it isn't 'smile' for you. You'll have to find your own 'you' thing. What I believe though, is that you can find your thing and then bring it into this practice. Move your you throughout your entire body. Move your you inside and out. Bring your you to everything with a sense of joy.

Allow yourself to be love.

By partaking in the practices and exercises in this book you're inviting self-love into the equation. Even reading through this book is allowing more self-love to surface. It's a daily choice, a continuous path- an evolution of love in practice.

Nursing from Within is about true, deep, and inner connection with the spirit of self. By reawakening your inner nurse with these inner shifts you embody the experience of nursing joy.

Each of us will walk our own path. It's been truly amazing to share these steps with you. Individually we strengthen and empower the nurse within; collectively we shift the entire profession of nursing

APPENDIX

Recommended Resources from Coaches, Teachers, Guides and Mentors:

Authentic Happiness: Using the New Positive Psychology to Realize Your Potential for Lasting Fulfillment by Martin E. P. Seligman

Awareness: The Perils and Opportunities of Reality by Anthony De Mello

Flow: The Psychology of Optimal Experience by Mihaly Csikszentmihalyi

Full Catastrophe Living by Jon Kabat-Zinn

Healing With Pleasure Medicine: PULSE by Coach Betty Louise

Journal to the Self: Twenty-Two Paths to Personal Growth by Kathleen Adams

Living the Reiki Way: Reiki Principles for Everyday Living by Penelope Quest

Reiki: A Comprehensive Guide by Pamela Miles

Reiki Energy Medicine: Bringing Healing Touch Into Home, Hospital, and Hospice by Libby Barnett, Maggie Babb and Susan Davidson

Reiki for the Heart and Soul: The Reiki Principles as Spiritual Pathwork by Amy Z. Rowland

The Artist's Way: A Spiritual Path to Higher Creativity by Julia Cameron

The Big Leap by Gay Hendricks

The Healing Consciousness: A Doctor's Journey to Healing by Beth Baughman DuPree

The Power of Patience: How this Old-Fashioned Virtue Can Improve Your Life by M.J. Ryan

The Secret of Deliberate Creation by Dr. Robert Anthony

The Untethered Soul: The Journey Beyond Yourself by Michael A. Singer

You Are More Than That: A Guide to Embracing the Spiritual Being Within and Becoming Fully Human by Rajiv Juneja M.D.

ABOUT THE AUTHOR

Spiritual Practice Nurse Elizabeth Scala is on a mission to shift the profession of nursing from the inside out.

Nurses typically enter their careers with a desire to provide compassionate, heart-based care. Challenged by regulations, financial pressures and technological advancements, todays nurse struggles to balance the art with the science of nursing.

As a speaker, author, workshop facilitator and retreat leader, Elizabeth inspires nursing teams to reconnect with the passionate and fulfilling joy that once called them to their roles.

In addition to this book, Elizabeth has written and published several others you may enjoy. These books include:

- Reiki Practice: A Nurse's Rx for Self-Care

- Bring Back the ART of Nursing: Reconnect to Your Nurse Within

- Learning through Experience: A Resource Book of Expert Interviews

- Back to the Basics: A Nurse's Pocket Guide to Self-Care

Elizabeth is also a certified coach and Reiki Master Teacher. She lives in Maryland with her supportive husband and playfully, silly pit bull. When Elizabeth's not speaking to or teaching other nurses you can find her enjoying nature, relaxing on the beach, doing Yoga or dancing to her favorite jam band, moe.

You can find out more about Elizabeth at **www.elizabethscala.com.**

BRING *NURSING FROM WITHIN* TO YOUR ORGANIZATION

In today's ever-changing, fast-paced healthcare environment, it is imperative that the profession of nursing stay ahead of the curve.

Nursing leadership often dreams of a staff that is satisfied, engaged and resilient yet far too often, competing priorities come into play. Heavy focus is given to patient safety, healthcare quality, and satisfaction measurements. Nurses are required to spend time and energy on policies and procedures, clinical informatics and regulatory affairs.

How can nursing staff stay engaged when the topic of 'resilience' gets quickly bumped from the agenda?

If you are a nurse leader who cares about the well-being of your staff, but feels guilty about the lack of time, capital or resources available- I am here to help!

Don't spend another sleepless night trying to figure out how 'fix' your nursing staff's teamwork and job satisfaction; I've got an easy, convenient and cost-effective answer for you.

Nursing from Within: An Rx for a Resilient and Healthy Team

As a motivational speaker, I can provide:

- Brief, on-the-go self-care touches for staff in the form of in-services, lunch-and-learns, or virtual webinars;

- More formal, yet highly engaging and inspirational presentations in the form of keynote speeches and convention program talks;

- Interactive, hands-on training in the form of half day seminars, full day workshops, or extended in-person retreats.

Contact Me to Get the Creative Juices Flowing Today:

(P): 410-929-0081

(E): support@elizabethscala.com

(L): www.linkedin.com/in/elizabethscala

(W): www.elizabethscala.com

Please Note: The 'Nursing from Within' complementary workbook, which will be chock full of self-reflective exercises, activity handouts and self-care tools will be available Spring, 2015. Check **www.elizabethscala.com** for details and to order then.

67347693R00080

Made in the USA
Lexington, KY
09 September 2017